AIR FRYER RECIPES 2021

DELICIOUS RECIPES FOR YOUR BREAKFAST TO BE MORE ENERGETIC

KIMBERLY SUTTON

Table of Contents

Introduction

Are you always looking for easier and more modern ways to cook the best meals for you and all your loved ones?
Are you constantly searching for useful kitchen appliances that will make your work in the kitchen more fun?
Well, you don't need to search anymore! We present to you today the best kitchen appliance available these days on the market: the air fryer!

Air fryers are simply the best kitchen tools for so many reasons. Are you interested in discovering more about air fryers? Then, pay attention next!

First of all, you need to know that air fryers are special and revolutionary kitchen appliances that cook your food using the circulation of hot air. These tools use a special technology called rapid air technology. Therefore, all the food you cook in these fryers is succulent on the inside and perfectly cooked on the outside.

The next thing you need to find out about air fryers is that they allow you to cook, bake, steam and roast pretty much everything you can imagine.

Last but not least, you should know that air fryers help you cook your meals in a much healthier way.
So many people all over the world just fell in love with this great and amazing tool and now it's your turn to become one of them.

So...long story short, we recommend you to purchase an air fryer right away and to get your hands on this cooking journal as soon as possible!

We can assure you that all the meals you cook in your air fryer will taste so good and that everyone will admire your cooking skills from now one!

So, let's get started!
Have fun cooking with your great air fryer!

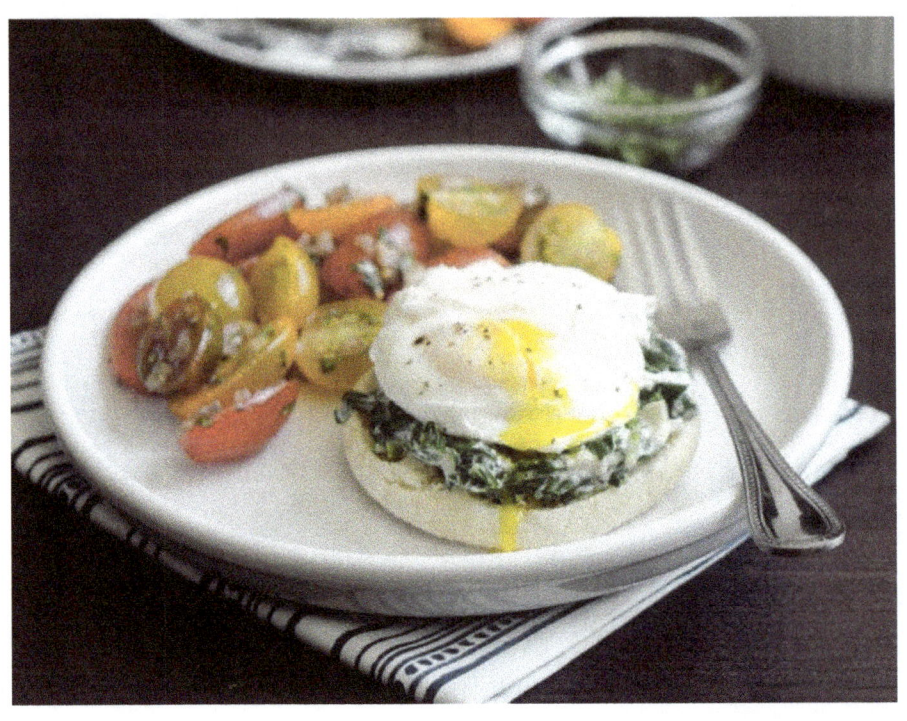

Air Fryer Breakfast Recipes

Tasty Baked Eggs

Preparation time: 10 minutes **Cooking time:** 20 minutes
Servings: 4

Ingredients:

- 4 eggs
- 1 pound baby spinach, torn
- 7 ounces ham, chopped
- 4 tablespoons milk
- 1 tablespoon olive oil
- Cooking spray
- Salt and black pepper to the taste

Directions:

1. Heat up a pan with the oil over medium heat, add baby spinach, stir cook for a couple of minutes and take off heat.
2. Grease 4 ramekins with cooking spray and divide baby spinach and ham in each.
3. Crack an egg in each ramekin, also divide milk, season with salt and pepper, place ramekins in

preheated air fryer at 350 degrees F and bake for 20 minutes.

4. Serve baked eggs for breakfast.

Enjoy!

Nutrition: calories 321, fat 6, fiber 8, carbs 15, protein 12

Breakfast Egg Bowls

Preparation time: 10 minutes **Cooking time:** 20 minutes
Servings: 4

Ingredients:

- 4 dinner rolls, tops cut off and insides scooped out
- 4 tablespoons heavy cream
- 4 eggs
- 4 tablespoons mixed chives and parsley
- Salt and black pepper to the taste
- 4 tablespoons parmesan, grated

Directions:

1. Arrange dinner rolls on a baking sheet and crack an egg in each.
2. Divide heavy cream, mixed herbs in each roll and season with salt and pepper.

3. Sprinkle parmesan on top of your rolls, place them in your air fryer and cook at 350 degrees F for 20 minutes.
4. Divide your bread bowls on plates and serve for breakfast.

Enjoy!

Nutrition: calories 238, fat 4, fiber 7, carbs 14, protein 7

Delicious Breakfast Soufflé

Preparation time: 10 minutes **Cooking time:** 8 minutes
Servings: 4

Ingredients:

- 4 eggs, whisked
- 4 tablespoons heavy cream
- A pinch of red chili pepper, crushed
- 2 tablespoons parsley, chopped
- 2 tablespoons chives, chopped
- Salt and black pepper to the taste

Directions:

1. In a bowl, mix eggs with salt, pepper, heavy cream, red chili pepper, parsley and chives, stir well and divide into 4 soufflé dishes.
2. Arrange dishes in your air fryer and cook soufflés at 350 degrees F for 8 minutes.
3. Serve them hot.

Enjoy!

Nutrition: calories 300, fat 7, fiber 9, carbs 15, protein 6

Air Fried Sandwich

Preparation time: 10 minutes **Cooking time:** 6 minutes
Servings: 2

Ingredients:

- 2 English muffins, halved
- 2 eggs
- 2 bacon strips
- Salt and black pepper to the taste

Directions:

1. Crack eggs in your air fryer, add bacon on top, cover and cook at 392 degrees F for 6 minutes.
2. Heat up your English muffin halves in your microwave for a few seconds, divide eggs on 2 halves, add bacon on top, season with salt and pepper, cover with the other 2 English muffins and serve for breakfast.

Enjoy!

Nutrition: calories 261, fat 5, fiber 8, carbs 12, protein 4

Rustic Breakfast

Preparation time: 10 minutes **Cooking time:** 13 minutes
Servings: 4

Ingredients:

- 7 ounces baby spinach
- 8 chestnuts mushrooms, halved
- 8 tomatoes, halved
- 1 garlic clove, minced
- 4 chipolatas
- 4 bacon slices, chopped
- Salt and black pepper to the taste
- 4 eggs
- Cooking spray

Directions:

1. Grease a cooking pan with the oil and add tomatoes, garlic and mushrooms.
2. Add bacon and chipolatas, also add spinach and crack eggs at the end.
3. Season with salt and pepper, place pan in the cooking basket of your air fryer and cook for 13 minutes at 350 degrees F.
4. Divide among plates and serve for breakfast.

Enjoy!

Nutrition: calories 312, fat 6, fiber 8, carbs 15, protein 5

Egg Muffins

Preparation time: 10 minutes **Cooking time:** 15 minutes
Servings: 4

Ingredients:

- 1 egg
- 2 tablespoons olive oil
- 3 tablespoons milk
- 3.5 ounces white flour
- 1 tablespoon baking powder
- 2 ounces parmesan, grated
- A splash of Worcestershire sauce

Directions:

1. In a bowl, mix egg with flour, oil, baking powder, milk, Worcestershire and parmesan, whisk well and divide into 4 silicon muffin cups.
2. Arrange cups in your air fryer's cooking basket, cover and cook at 392, degrees F for 15 minutes.
3. Serve warm for breakfast.

Enjoy!

Nutrition: calories 251, fat 6, fiber 8, carbs 9, protein 3

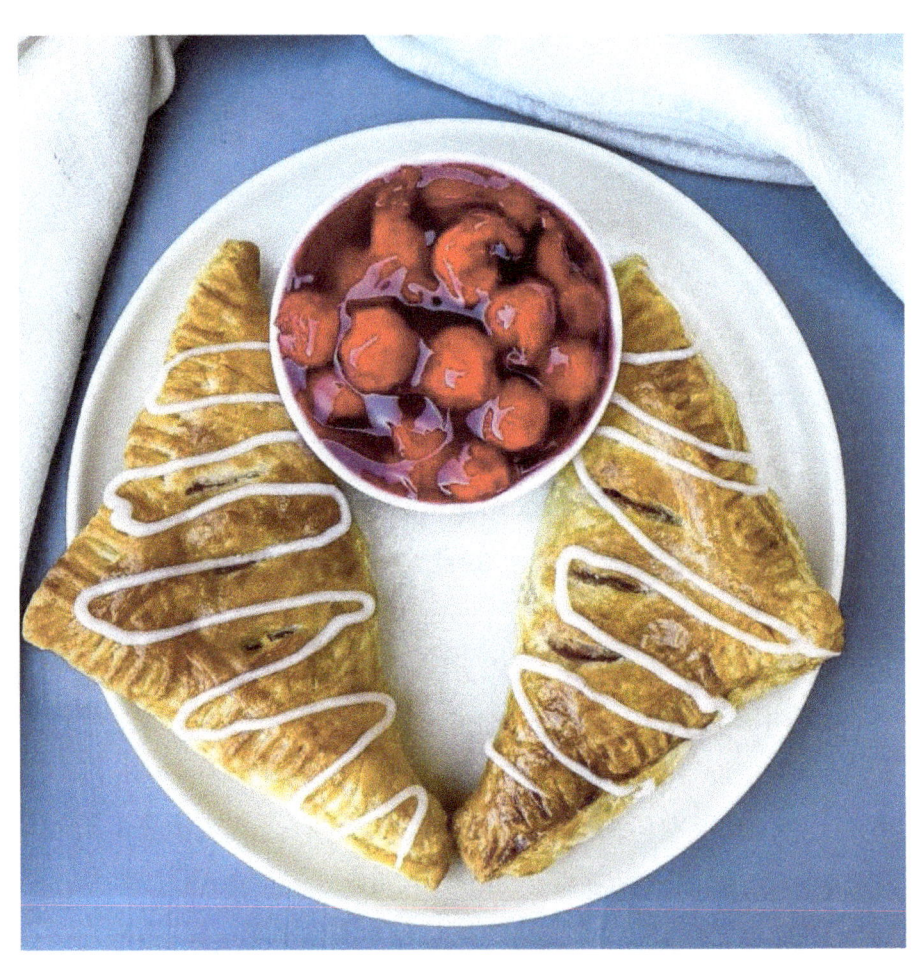

Polenta Bites

Preparation time: 10 minutes **Cooking time:** 20 minutes
Servings: 4

Ingredients:

For the polenta:

- 1 tablespoon butter
- 1 cup cornmeal
- 3 cups water
- Salt and black pepper to the taste

For the polenta bites:

- 2 tablespoons powdered sugar
- Cooking spray

Directions:

1. In a pan, mix water with cornmeal, butter, salt and pepper, stir, bring to a boil over medium heat, cook for 10 minutes, take off heat, whisk one more time and keep in the fridge until it's cold.
2. Scoop 1 tablespoon of polenta, shape a ball and place on a working surface.
3. Repeat with the rest of the polenta, arrange all the balls in the cooking basket of your air fryer, spray them with cooking spray, cover and cook at 380 degrees F for 8 minutes.
4. Arrange polenta bites on plates, sprinkle sugar all over and serve for breakfast.

Enjoy!

Nutrition: calories 231, fat 7, fiber 8, carbs 12, protein 4

Delicious Breakfast Potatoes

Preparation time: 10 minutes **Cooking time:** 35 minutes
Servings: 4

Ingredients:

- 2 tablespoons olive oil
- 3 potatoes, cubed
- 1 yellow onion, chopped
- 1 red bell pepper, chopped
- Salt and black pepper to the taste
- 1 teaspoon garlic powder
- 1 teaspoon sweet paprika
- 1 teaspoon onion powder

Directions:

1. Grease your air fryer's basket with olive oil, add potatoes, toss and season with salt and pepper.
2. Add onion, bell pepper, garlic powder, paprika and onion powder, toss well, cover and cook at 370 degrees F for 30 minutes.
3. Divide potatoes mix on plates and serve for breakfast.

Enjoy!

Nutrition: calories 214, fat 6, fiber 8, carbs 15, protein 4

Tasty Cinnamon Toast

Preparation time: 10 minutes **Cooking time:** 5 minutes
Servings: 6

Ingredients:

- 1 stick butter, soft
- 12 bread slices
- ½ cup sugar
- 1 and ½ teaspoon vanilla extract
- 1 and ½ teaspoon cinnamon powder

Directions:

1. In a bowl, mix soft butter with sugar, vanilla and cinnamon and whisk well.
2. Spread this on bread slices, place them in your air fryer and cook at 400 degrees F for 5 minutes,
3. Divide among plates and serve for breakfast.

Enjoy!

Nutrition: calories 221, fat 4, fiber 7, carbs 12, protein 8

Delicious Potato Hash

Preparation time: 10 minutes **Cooking time:** 25 minutes
Servings: 4

Ingredients:
- 1 and ½ potatoes, cubed
- 1 yellow onion, chopped
- 2 teaspoons olive oil
- 1 green bell pepper, chopped
- Salt and black pepper to the taste
- ½ teaspoon thyme, dried
- 2 eggs

Directions:
1. Heat up your air fryer at 350 degrees F, add oil, heat it up, add onion, bell pepper, salt and pepper, stir and cook for 5 minutes.
2. Add potatoes, thyme and eggs, stir, cover and cook at 360 degrees F for 20 minutes.
3. Divide among plates and serve for breakfast.

Enjoy!

Nutrition: calories 241, fat 4, fiber 7, carbs 12, protein 7

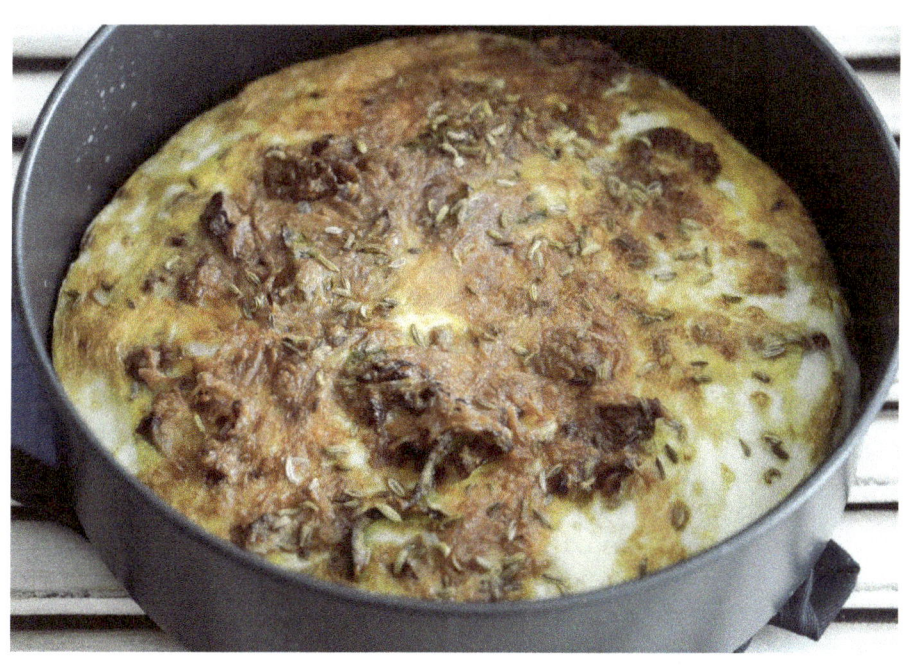

Sweet Breakfast Casserole

Preparation time: 10 minutes **Cooking time:** 30 minutes
Servings: 4

Ingredients:

- 3 tablespoons brown sugar
- 4 tablespoons butter
- 2 tablespoons white sugar
- ½ teaspoon cinnamon powder
- ½ cup flour

For the casserole:

- 2 eggs
- 2 tablespoons white sugar
- 2 and ½ cups white flour
- 1 teaspoon baking soda
- 1 teaspoon baking powder
- 2 eggs
- ½ cup milk
- 2 cups buttermilk
- 4 tablespoons butter
- Zest from 1 lemon, grated
- 1 and 2/3 cup blueberries

Directions:

1. In a bowl, mix eggs with 2 tablespoons white sugar, 2 and ½ cups white flour, baking powder, baking soda, 2 eggs, milk, buttermilk, 4 tablespoons butter, lemon zest and blueberries, stir and pour into a pan that fits your air fryer.
2. In another bowls, mix 3 tablespoons brown sugar with 2 tablespoons white sugar, 4 tablespoons butter, ½ cup flour and cinnamon, stir until you obtain a crumble and spread over blueberries mix.
3. Place in preheated air fryer and bake at 300 degrees F for 30 minutes.
4. Divide among plates and serve for breakfast.

Enjoy!

Nutrition: calories 214, fat 5, fiber 8, carbs 12, protein 5

Eggs Casserole

Preparation time: 10 minutes **Cooking time:** 25 minutes
Servings: 6

Ingredients:
- 1 pound turkey, ground
- 1 tablespoon olive oil
- ½ teaspoon chili powder
- 12 eggs
- 1 sweet potato, cubed
- 1 cup baby spinach
- Salt and black pepper to the taste
- 2 tomatoes, chopped for serving

Directions:
1. In a bowl, mix eggs with salt, pepper, chili powder, potato, spinach, turkey and sweet potato and whisk well.
2. Heat up your air fryer at 350 degrees F, add oil and heat it up.

3. Add eggs mix, spread into your air fryer, cover and cook for 25 minutes.

4. Divide among plates and serve for breakfast.

Enjoy!

Nutrition: calories 300, fat 5, fiber 8, carbs 13, protein 6

Sausage, Eggs and Cheese Mix

Preparation time: 10 minutes **Cooking time:** 20 minutes
Servings: 4

Ingredients:

- 10 ounces sausages, cooked and crumbled
- 1 cup cheddar cheese, shredded
- 1 cup mozzarella cheese, shredded
- 8 eggs, whisked
- 1 cup milk
- Salt and black pepper to the taste
- Cooking spray

Directions:

1. In a bowl, mix sausages with cheese, mozzarella, eggs, milk, salt and pepper and whisk well.
2. Heat up your air fryer at 380 degrees F, spray cooking oil, add eggs and sausage mix and cook for 20 minutes.
3. Divide among plates and serve.

Enjoy!

Nutrition: calories 320, fat 6, fiber 8, carbs 12, protein 5

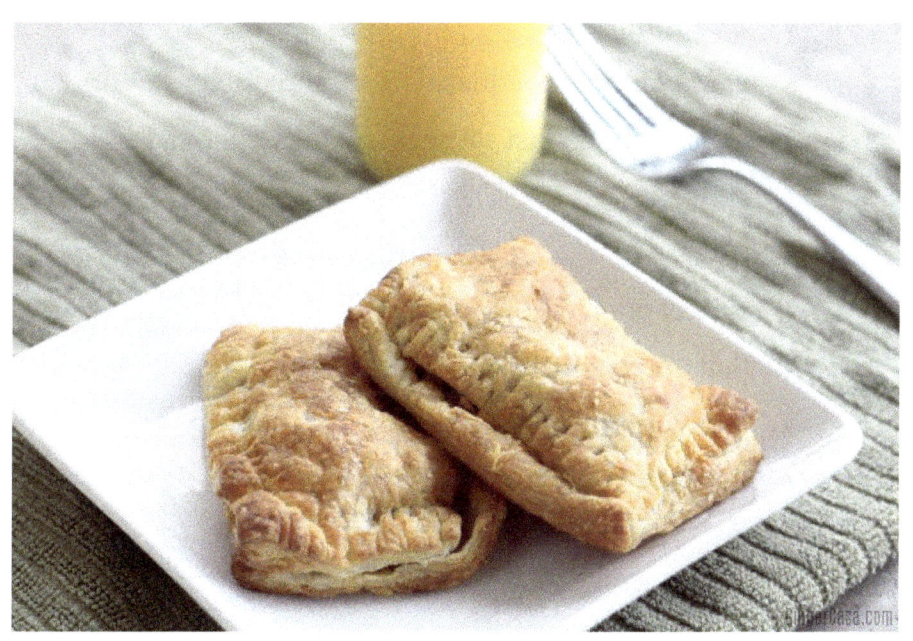

Cheese Air Fried Bake

Preparation time: 10 minutes **Cooking time:** 20 minutes
Servings: 4

Ingredients:

- 4 bacon slices, cooked and crumbled
- 2 cups milk
- 2 and ½ cups cheddar cheese, shredded
- 1 pound breakfast sausage, casings removed and chopped
- 2 eggs
- ½ teaspoon onion powder
- Salt and black pepper to the taste
- 3 tablespoons parsley, chopped
- Cooking spray

Directions:

1. In a bowl, mix eggs with milk, cheese, onion powder, salt, pepper and parsley and whisk well.
2. Grease your air fryer with cooking spray, heat it up at 320 degrees F and add bacon and sausage.
3. Add eggs mix, spread and cook for 20 minutes.
4. Divide among plates and serve.

Enjoy!

Nutrition: calories 214, fat 5, fiber 8, carbs 12, protein 12

Biscuits Casserole

Preparation time: 10 minutes **Cooking time:** 15 minutes
Servings: 8

Ingredients:

- 12 ounces biscuits, quartered
- 3 tablespoons flour
- ½ pound sausage, chopped
- A pinch of salt and black pepper
- 2 and ½ cups milk
- Cooking spray

Directions:

1. Grease your air fryer with cooking spray and heat it over 350 degrees F.
2. Add biscuits on the bottom and mix with sausage.
3. Add flour, milk, salt and pepper, toss a bit and cook for 15 minutes.
4. Divide among plates and serve for breakfast.

Enjoy!

Nutrition: calories 321, fat 4, fiber 7, carbs 12, protein 5

Turkey Burrito

Preparation time: 10 minutes **Cooking time:** 10 minutes
Servings: 2

Ingredients:
- 4 slices turkey breast already cooked
- ½ red bell pepper, sliced
- 2 eggs
- 1 small avocado, peeled, pitted and sliced
- 2 tablespoons salsa
- Salt and black pepper to the taste
- 1/8 cup mozzarella cheese, grated
- Tortillas for serving

Directions:
1. In a bowl, whisk eggs with salt and pepper to the taste, pour them in a pan and place it in the air fryer's basket.
2. Cook at 400 degrees F for 5 minutes, take pan out of the fryer and transfer eggs to a plate.

3. Arrange tortillas on a working surface, divide eggs on them, also divide turkey meat, bell pepper, cheese, salsa and avocado.
4. Roll your burritos and place them in your air fryer after you've lined it with some tin foil.
5. Heat up the burritos at 300 degrees F for 3 minutes, divide them on plates and serve.

Enjoy!

Nutrition: calories 349, fat 23, fiber 11, carbs 20, protein 21

Tofu Scramble

Preparation time: 5 minutes **Cooking time:** 30 minutes
Servings: 4

Ingredients:

- 2 tablespoons soy sauce
- 1 tofu block, cubed
- 1 teaspoon turmeric, ground
- 2 tablespoons extra virgin olive oil
- 4 cups broccoli florets
- ½ teaspoon onion powder
- ½ teaspoon garlic powder
- 2 and ½ cup red potatoes, cubed
- ½ cup yellow onion, chopped
- Salt and black pepper to the taste

Directions:

1. Mix tofu with 1 tablespoon oil, salt, pepper, soy sauce, garlic powder, onion powder, turmeric and onion in a bowl, stir and leave aside.
2. In a separate bowl, combine potatoes with the rest of the oil, a pinch of salt and pepper and toss to coat.

3. Put potatoes in your air fryer at 350 degrees F and bake for 15 minutes, shaking once.
4. Add tofu and its marinade to your air fryer and bake for 15 minutes.
5. Add broccoli to the fryer and cook everything for 5 minutes more.
6. Serve right away.

Enjoy!

Nutrition: calories 140, fat 4, fiber 3, carbs 10, protein 14

Oatmeal Casserole

Preparation time: 10 minutes **Cooking time:** 20 minutes
Servings: 8

Ingredients:

- 2 cups rolled oats
- 1 teaspoon baking powder
- 1/3 cup brown sugar
- 1 teaspoon cinnamon powder
- ½ cup chocolate chips
- 2/3 cup blueberries
- 1 banana, peeled and mashed
- 2 cups milk
- 1 eggs
- 2 tablespoons butter
- 1 teaspoon vanilla extract
- Cooking spray

Directions:

1. In a bowl, mix sugar with baking powder, cinnamon, chocolate chips, blueberries and banana and stir.
2. In a separate bowl, mix eggs with vanilla extract and butter and stir.

3. Heat up your air fryer at 320 degrees F, grease with cooking spray and add oats on the bottom.
4. Add cinnamon mix and eggs mix, toss and cook for 20 minutes.
5. Stir one more time, divide into bowls and serve for breakfast.

Enjoy!

Nutrition: calories 300, fat 4, fiber 7, carbs 12, protein 10

Ham Breakfast

Preparation time: 10 minutes **Cooking time:** 15 minutes
Servings: 6

Ingredients:

- 6 cups French bread, cubed
- 4 ounces green chilies, chopped
- 10 ounces ham, cubed
- 4 ounces cheddar cheese, shredded
- 2 cups milk
- 5 eggs
- 1 tablespoon mustard
- Salt and black pepper to the taste
- Cooking spray

Directions:

1. Heat up your air fryer at 350 degrees F and grease it with cooking spray.
2. In a bowl, mix eggs with milk, cheese, mustard, salt and pepper and stir.
3. Add bread cubes in your air fryer and mix with chilies and ham.
4. Add eggs mix, spread and cook for 15 minutes.
5. Divide among plates and serve.

Enjoy!

Nutrition: calories 200, fat 5, fiber 6, carbs 12, protein 14

Tomato and Bacon Breakfast

Preparation time: 10 minutes **Cooking time:** 30 minutes
Servings: 6

Ingredients:

- 1 pound white bread, cubed
- 1 pound smoked bacon, cooked and chopped
- ¼ cup olive oil
- 1 yellow onion, chopped
- 28 ounces canned tomatoes, chopped
- ½ teaspoon red pepper, crushed
- ½ pound cheddar, shredded
- 2 tablespoons chives, chopped
- ½ pound Monterey jack, shredded
- 2 tablespoons stock
- Salt and black pepper to the taste
- 8 eggs, whisked

Directions:

1. Add the oil to your air fryer and heat it up at 350 degrees F.
2. Add bread, bacon, onion, tomatoes, red pepper and stock and stir.
3. Add eggs, cheddar and Monterey jack and cook everything for 20 minutes.
4. Divide among plates, sprinkle chives and serve.

Enjoy!

Nutrition: calories 231, fat 5, fiber 7, carbs 12, protein 4

Tasty Hash

Preparation time: 10 minutes **Cooking time:** 15 minutes
Servings: 6

Ingredients:

- 16 ounces hash browns
- ¼ cup olive oil
- ½ teaspoon paprika
- ½ teaspoon garlic powder
- Salt and black pepper to the taste
- 1 egg, whisked
- 2 tablespoon chives, chopped
- 1 cup cheddar, shredded

Directions:

1. Add oil to your air fryer, heat it up at 350 degrees F and add hash browns.
2. Also add paprika, garlic powder, salt, pepper and egg, toss and cook for 15 minutes.
3. Add cheddar and chives, toss, divide among plates and serve.

Enjoy!

Nutrition: calories 213, fat 7, fiber 8, carbs 12, protein 4

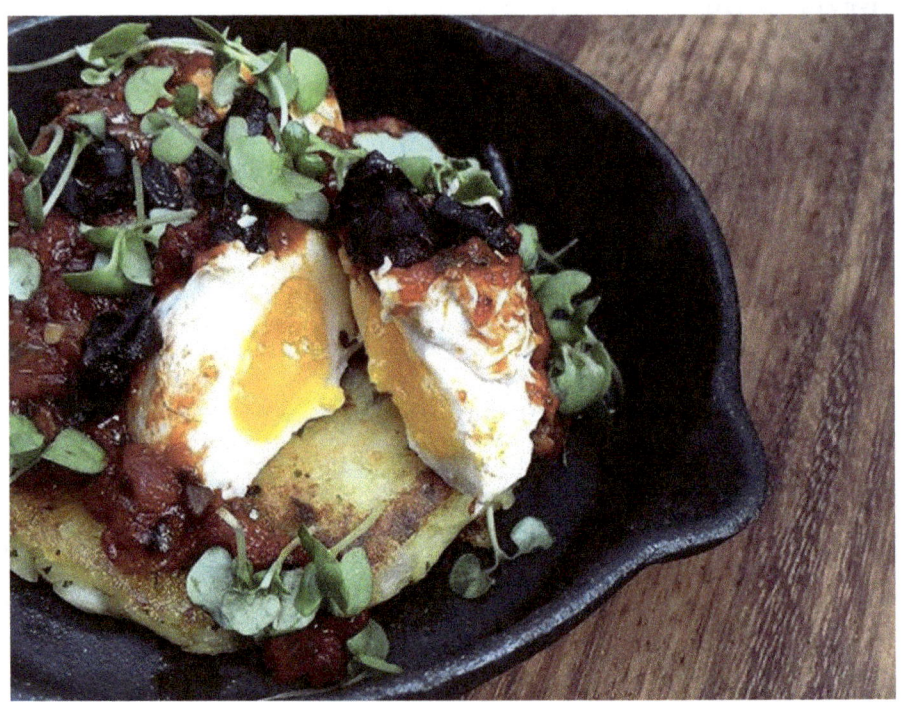

Creamy Hash Browns

Preparation time: 10 minutes **Cooking time:** 20 minutes
Servings: 6

Ingredients:

- 2 pounds hash browns
- 1 cup whole milk
- 8 bacon slices, chopped
- 9 ounces cream cheese
- 1 yellow onion, chopped
- 1 cup cheddar cheese, shredded
- 6 green onions, chopped
- Salt and black pepper to the taste
- 6 eggs
- Cooking spray

Directions:

1. Heat up your air fryer at 350 degrees F and grease it with cooking spray.
2. In a bowl, mix eggs with milk, cream cheese, cheddar cheese, bacon, onion, salt and pepper and whisk well.
3. Add hash browns to your air fryer, add eggs mix over them and cook for 20 minutes.
4. Divide among plates and serve.

Enjoy!

Nutrition: calories 261, fat 6, fiber 9, carbs 8, protein 12

Blackberry French Toast

Preparation time: 10 minutes **Cooking time:** 20 minutes
Servings: 6

Ingredients:

- 1 cup blackberry jam, warm
- 12 ounces bread loaf, cubed
- 8 ounces cream cheese, cubed
- 4 eggs
- 1 teaspoon cinnamon powder
- 2 cups half and half
- ½ cup brown sugar
- 1 teaspoon vanilla extract
- Cooking spray

Directions:

1. Grease your air fryer with cooking spray and heat it up at 300 degrees F.
2. Add blueberry jam on the bottom, layer half of the bread cubes, then add cream cheese and top with the rest of the bread.
3. In a bowl, mix eggs with half and half, cinnamon, sugar and vanilla, whisk well and add over bread mix.
4. Cook for 20 minutes, divide among plates and serve for breakfast.

Enjoy!

Nutrition: calories 215, fat 6, fiber 9, carbs 16, protein 6

Smoked Sausage Breakfast Mix

Preparation time: 10 minutes **Cooking time:** 30 minutes
Servings: 4

Ingredients:

- 1 and ½ pounds smoked sausage, chopped and browned
- A pinch of salt and black pepper
- 1 and ½ cups grits
- 4 and ½ cups water
- 16 ounces cheddar cheese, shredded
- 1 cup milk
- ¼ teaspoon garlic powder
- 1 and ½ teaspoons thyme, chopped
- Cooking spray
- 4 eggs, whisked

Directions:

1. Put the water in a pot, bring to a boil over medium heat, add grits, stir, cover, cook for 5 minutes and take off heat.

2. Add cheese, stir until it melts and mix with milk, thyme, salt, pepper, garlic powder and eggs and whisk really well.
3. Heat up your air fryer at 300 degrees F, grease with cooking spray and add browned sausage.
4. Add grits mix, spread and cook for 25 minutes.
5. Divide among plates and serve for breakfast.

Enjoy!

Nutrition: calories 321, fat 6, fiber 7, carbs 17, protein 4

Delicious Potato Frittata

Preparation time: 10 minutes **Cooking time:** 20 minutes
Servings: 6

Ingredients:

- 6 ounces jarred roasted red bell peppers, chopped
- 12 eggs, whisked
- ½ cup parmesan, grated
- 3 garlic cloves, minced
- 2 tablespoons parsley, chopped
- Salt and black pepper to the taste
- 2 tablespoons chives, chopped
- 16 potato wedges
- 6 tablespoons ricotta cheese
- Cooking spray

Directions:

1. In a bowl, mix eggs with red peppers, garlic, parsley, salt, pepper and ricotta and whisk well.
2. Heat up your air fryer at 300 degrees F and grease it with cooking spray.
3. Add half of the potato wedges on the bottom and sprinkle half of the parmesan all over.

4. Add half of the egg mix, add the rest of the potatoes and the rest of the parmesan.
5. Add the rest of the eggs mix, sprinkle chives and cook for 20 minutes.
6. Divide among plates and serve for breakfast.

Enjoy!

Nutrition: calories 312, fat 6, fiber 9, carbs 16, protein 5

Asparagus Frittata

Preparation time: 10 minutes **Cooking time:** 5 minutes
Servings: 2

Ingredients:

- 4 eggs, whisked
- 2 tablespoons parmesan, grated
- 4 tablespoons milk
- Salt and black pepper to the taste
- 10 asparagus tips, steamed
- Cooking spray

Directions:

1. In a bowl, mix eggs with parmesan, milk, salt and pepper and whisk well.
2. Heat up your air fryer at 400 degrees F and grease with cooking spray.
3. Add asparagus, add eggs mix, toss a bit and cook for 5 minutes.
4. Divide frittata on plates and serve for breakfast.

Enjoy!

Nutrition: calories 312, fat 5, fiber 8, carbs 14, protein 2

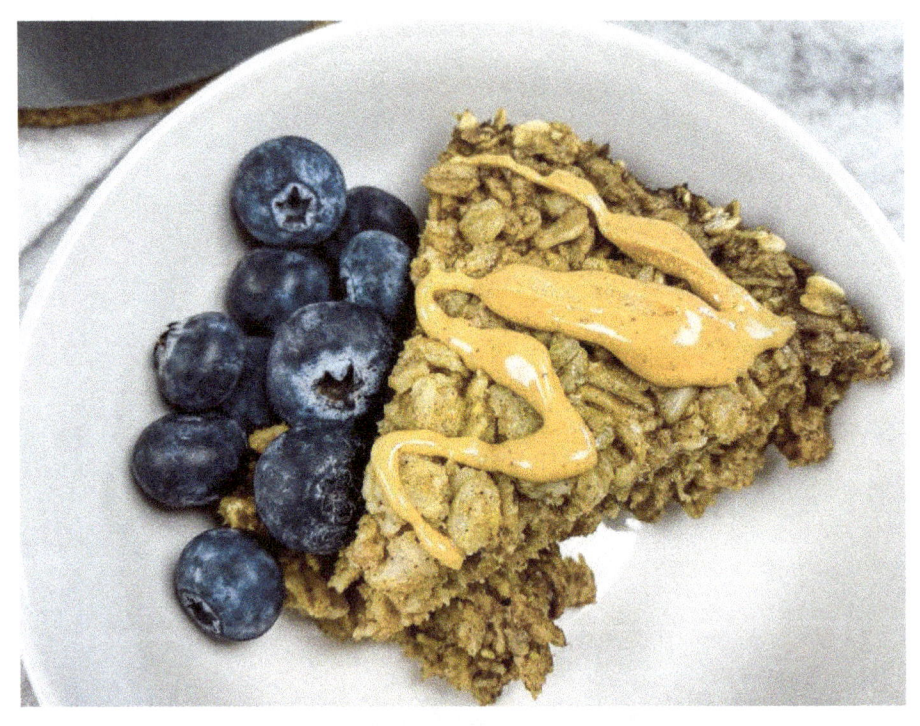

Special Corn Flakes Breakfast Casserole

Preparation time: 10 minutes **Cooking time:** 8 minutes
Servings: 5

Ingredients:

- 1/3 cup milk
- 3 teaspoons sugar
- 2 eggs, whisked
- ¼ teaspoon nutmeg, ground
- ¼ cup blueberries
- 4 tablespoons cream cheese, whipped
- 1 and ½ cups corn flakes, crumbled
- 5 bread slices

Directions:

1. In a bowl, mix eggs with sugar, nutmeg and milk and whisk well.
2. In another bowl, mix cream cheese with blueberries and whisk well.
3. Put corn flakes in a third bowl.
4. Spread blueberry mix on each bread slice, then dip in eggs mix and dredge in corn flakes at the end.

5. Place bread in your air fryer's basket, heat up at 400 degrees F and bake for 8 minutes.
6. Divide among plates and serve for breakfast.

Enjoy!

Nutrition: calories 300, fat 5, fiber 7, carbs 16, protein 4

Ham Breakfast Pie

Preparation time: 10 minutes **Cooking time:** 25 minutes
Servings: 6

Ingredients:

- 16 ounces crescent rolls dough
- 2 eggs, whisked
- 2 cups cheddar cheese, grated
- 1 tablespoon parmesan, grated
- 2 cups ham, cooked and chopped
- Salt and black pepper to the taste
- Cooking spray

Directions:

1. Grease your air fryer's pan with cooking spray and press half of the crescent rolls dough on the bottom.
2. In a bowl, mix eggs with cheddar cheese, parmesan, salt and pepper, whisk well and add over dough.
3. Spread ham, cut the rest of the crescent rolls dough in strips, arrange them over ham and cook at 300 degrees F for 25 minutes.
4. Slice pie and serve for breakfast.

Enjoy!

Nutrition: calories 400, fat 27, fiber 7, carbs 22, protein 16

Breakfast Veggie Mix

Preparation time: 10 minutes **Cooking time:** 25 minutes
Servings: 6

Ingredients:

- 1 yellow onion, sliced
- 1 red bell pepper, chopped
- 1 gold potato, chopped
- 2 tablespoons olive oil
- 8 ounces brie, trimmed and cubed
- 12 ounces sourdough bread, cubed
- 4 ounces parmesan, grated
- 8 eggs
- 2 tablespoons mustard
- 3 cups milk
- Salt and black pepper to the taste

Directions:

1. Heat up your air fryer at 350 degrees F, add oil, onion, potato and bell pepper and cook for 5 minutes.
2. In a bowl, mix eggs with milk, salt, pepper and mustard and whisk well.

3. Add bread and brie to your air fryer, add half of the eggs mix and add half of the parmesan as well.
4. Add the rest of the bread and parmesan, toss just a little bit and cook for 20 minutes.
5. Divide among plates and serve for breakfast.

Enjoy!

Nutrition: calories 231, fat 5, fiber 10, carbs 20, protein 12

Scrambled Eggs

Preparation time: 10 minutes **Cooking time:** 10 minutes
Servings: 2

Ingredients:

- 2 eggs
- 2 tablespoons butter
- Salt and black pepper to the taste
- 1 red bell pepper, chopped
- A pinch of sweet paprika

Directions:

1. In a bowl, mix eggs with salt, pepper, paprika and red bell pepper and whisk well.
2. Heat up your air fryer at 140 degrees F, add butter and melt it.
3. Add eggs mix, stir and cook for 10 minutes.
4. Divide scrambled eggs on plates and serve for breakfast.

Enjoy!

Nutrition: calories 200, fat 4, fiber 7, carbs 10, protein 3

Fast Eggs and Tomatoes

Preparation time: 5 minutes **Cooking time:** 10 minutes
Servings: 4

Ingredients:

- 4 eggs
- 2 ounces milk
- 2 tablespoons parmesan, grated
- Salt and black pepper to the taste
- 8 cherry tomatoes, halved
- Cooking spray

Directions:

1. Grease your air fryer with cooking spray and heat it up at 200 degrees F.
2. In a bowl, mix eggs with cheese, milk, salt and pepper and whisk.
3. Add this mix to your air fryer and cook for 6 minutes.
4. Add tomatoes, cook your scrambled eggs for 3 minutes, divide among plates and serve.

Enjoy!

Nutrition: calories 200, fat 4, fiber 7, carbs 12, protein 3

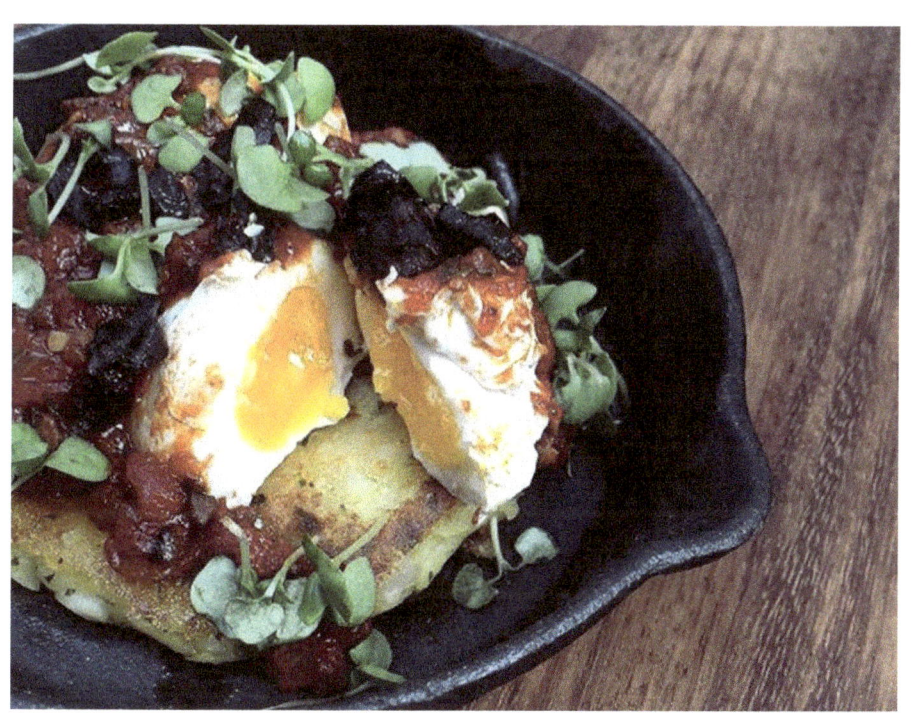

Air Fried Tomato Breakfast Quiche

Preparation time: 10 minutes **Cooking time:** 30 minutes
Servings: 1

Ingredients:

- 2 tablespoons yellow onion, chopped
- 2 eggs
- ¼ cup milk
- ½ cup gouda cheese, shredded
- ¼ cup tomatoes, chopped
- Salt and black pepper to the taste
- Cooking spray

Directions:

1. Grease a ramekin with cooking spray.
2. Crack eggs, add onion, milk, cheese, tomatoes, salt and pepper and stir.
3. Add this in your air fryer's pan and cook at 340 degrees F for 30 minutes.
4. Serve hot.

Enjoy!

Nutrition: calories 241, fat 6, fiber 8, carbs 14, protein 6

Breakfast Mushroom Quiche

Preparation time: 10 minutes **Cooking time:** 10 minutes
Servings: 4

Ingredients:

- 1 tablespoon flour
- 1 tablespoon butter, soft
- 9 inch pie dough
- 2 button mushrooms, chopped
- 2 tablespoons ham, chopped
- 3 eggs
- 1 small yellow onion, chopped
- 1/3 cup heavy cream
- A pinch of nutmeg, ground
- Salt and black pepper to the taste
- ½ teaspoon thyme, dried
- ¼ cup Swiss cheese, grated

Directions:

1. Dust a working surface with the flour and roll the pie dough.
2. Press in on the bottom of the pie pan your air fryer has.

3. In a bowl, mix butter with mushrooms, ham, onion, eggs, heavy cream, salt, pepper, thyme and nutmeg and whisk well.
4. Add this over pie crust, spread, sprinkle Swiss cheese all over and place pie pan in your air fryer.
5. Cook your quiche at 400 degrees F for 10 minutes.
6. Slice and serve for breakfast.

Enjoy!

Nutrition: calories 212, fat 4, fiber 6, carbs 7, protein 7

Smoked Air Fried Tofu Breakfast

Preparation time: 10 minutes **Cooking time:** 12 minutes
Servings: 2

Ingredients:

- 1 tofu block, pressed and cubed
- Salt and black pepper to the taste
- 1 tablespoon smoked paprika
- ¼ cup cornstarch
- Cooking spray

Directions:

1. Grease your air fryer's basket with cooking spray and heat the fryer at 370 degrees F.
2. In a bowl, mix tofu with salt, pepper, smoked paprika and cornstarch and toss well.
3. Add tofu to you air fryer's basket and cook for 12 minutes shaking the fryer every 4 minutes.
4. Divide into bowls and serve for breakfast.

Enjoy!

Nutrition: calories 172, fat 4, fiber 7, carbs 12, protein 4

Delicious Tofu and Mushrooms

Preparation time: 10 minutes **Cooking time:** 10 minutes
Servings: 2

Ingredients:

- 1 tofu block, pressed and cut into medium pieces
- 1 cup panko bread crumbs
- Salt and black pepper to the taste
- ½ tablespoons flour
- 1 egg
- 1 tablespoon mushrooms, minced

Directions:

1. In a bowl, mix egg with mushrooms, flour, salt and pepper and whisk well.
2. Dip tofu pieces in egg mix, then dredge them in panko bread crumbs, place them in your air fryer and cook at 350 degrees F for 10 minutes.
3. Serve them for breakfast right away.

Enjoy!

Nutrition: calories 142, fat 4, fiber 6, carbs 8, protein 3

Breakfast Broccoli Quiche

Preparation time: 10 minutes **Cooking time:** 20 minutes
Servings: 2

Ingredients:

- 1 broccoli head, florets separated and steamed
- 1 tomato, chopped
- 3 carrots, chopped and steamed
- 2 ounces cheddar cheese, grated
- 2 eggs
- 2 ounces milk
- 1 teaspoon parsley, chopped
- 1 teaspoon thyme, chopped
- Salt and black pepper to the taste

Directions:

1. In a bowl, mix eggs with milk, parsley, thyme, salt and pepper and whisk well.
2. Put broccoli, carrots and tomato in your air fryer.
3. Add eggs mix on top, spread cheddar cheese, cover and cook at 350 degrees F for 20 minutes.
4. Divide among plates and serve for breakfast.

Enjoy!

Nutrition: calories 214, fat 4, fiber 7, carbs 12, protein 3

Creamy Eggs

Preparation time: 10 minutes **Cooking time:** 12 minutes
Servings: 4

Ingredients:

- 2 teaspoons butter, soft
- 2 ham slices
- 4 eggs
- 2 tablespoons heavy cream
- Salt and black pepper to the taste
- 3 tablespoons parmesan, grated
- 2 teaspoons chives, chopped
- A pinch of smoked paprika

Directions:

1. Grease your air fryer's pan with the butter, line it with the ham and add it to your air fryer's basket.
2. In a bowl, mix 1 egg with heavy cream, salt and pepper, whisk well and add over ham.
3. Crack the rest of the eggs in the pan, sprinkle parmesan and cook your mix for 12 minutes at 320 degrees F.

4. Sprinkle paprika and chives all over, divide among plates and serve for breakfast.

Enjoy!

Nutrition: calories 263, fat 5, fiber 8, carbs 12, protein 5

Cheesy Breakfast Bread

Preparation time: 10 minutes **Cooking time:** 8 minutes
Servings: 3

Ingredients:

- 6 bread slices
- 5 tablespoons butter, melted
- 3 garlic cloves, minced
- 6 teaspoons sun dried tomato pesto
- 1 cup mozzarella cheese, grated

Directions:

1. Arrange bread slices on a working surface.
2. Spread butter all over, divide tomato paste, garlic and top with grated cheese.
3. Add bread slices to your heated air fryer and cook them at 350 degrees F for 8 minutes.
4. Divide among plates and serve for breakfast.

Enjoy!

Nutrition: calories 187, fat 5, fiber 6, carbs 8, protein 3

Breakfast Bread Pudding

Preparation time: 10 minutes **Cooking time:** 22 minutes
Servings: 4

Ingredients:

- ½ pound white bread, cubed
- ¾ cup milk
- ¾ cup water
- 2 teaspoons cornstarch
- ½ cup apple, peeled, cored and roughly chopped
- 5 tablespoons honey
- 1 teaspoon vanilla extract
- 2 teaspoons cinnamon powder
- 1 and 1/3 cup flour
- 3/5 cup brown sugar
- 3 ounces soft butter

Directions:

1. In a bowl, mix bread with apple, milk with water, honey, cinnamon, vanilla and cornstarch and whisk well.
2. In a separate bowl, mix flour with sugar and butter and stir until you obtain a crumbled mixture.

3. Press half of the crumble mix on the bottom of your air fryer, add bread and apple mix, add the rest of the crumble and cook everything at 350 degrees F for 22 minutes.
4. Divide bread pudding on plates and serve.

Enjoy!

Nutrition: calories 261, fat 7, fiber 7, carbs 8, protein 5

Buttermilk Breakfast Biscuits

Preparation time: 10 minutes **Cooking time:** 8 minutes
Servings: 4

Ingredients:

- 1 and ¼ cup white flour
- ½ cup self-rising flour
- ¼ teaspoon baking soda
- ½ teaspoon baking powder
- 1 teaspoon sugar
- 4 tablespoons butter, cold and cubed+ 1 tablespoon melted butter
- ¾ cup buttermilk
- Maple syrup for serving

Directions:

1. In a bowl, mix white flour with self-rising flour, baking soda, baking powder and sugar and stir.
2. Add cold butter and stir using your hands.
3. Add buttermilk, stir until you obtain a dough and transfer to a floured working surface.
4. Roll your dough and cut 10 pieces using a round cutter.

5. Arrange biscuits in your air fryer's cake pan, brush them with melted butter and cook at 400 degrees F for 8 minutes.

6. Serve them for breakfast with some maple syrup on top.

Enjoy!

Nutrition: calories 192, fat 6, fiber 9, carbs 12, protein 3

Breakfast Bread Rolls

Preparation time: 10 minutes **Cooking time:** 12 minutes
Servings: 4

Ingredients:

- 5 potatoes, boiled, peeled and mashed
- 8 bread slices, white parts only
- 1 coriander bunch, chopped
- 2 green chilies, chopped
- 2 small yellow onions, chopped
- ½ teaspoon turmeric powder
- 2 curry leaf springs
- ½ teaspoon mustard seeds
- 2 tablespoons olive oil
- Salt and black pepper to the taste

Directions:

1. Heat up a pan with 1 teaspoon oil, add mustard seeds, onions, curry leaves and turmeric, stir and cook for a few seconds.
2. Add mashed potatoes, salt, pepper, coriander and chilies, stir well, take off heat and cool it down.

3. Divide potatoes mix into 8 parts and shape ovals using your wet hands.
4. Wet bread slices with water, press in order to drain excess water and keep one slice in your palm.
5. Add a potato oval over bread slice and wrap it around it.
6. Repeat with the rest of the potato mix and bread.
7. Heat up your air fryer at 400 degrees F, add the rest of the oil, add bread rolls, cook them for 12 minutes.
8. Divide bread rolls on plates and serve for breakfast.

Enjoy!

Nutrition: calories 261, fat 6, fiber 9, carbs 12, protein 7

Spanish Omelet

Preparation time: 10 minutes **Cooking time:** 10 minutes
Servings: 4

Ingredients:

- 3 eggs
- ½ chorizo, chopped
- 1 potato, peeled and cubed
- ½ cup corn
- 1 tablespoon olive oil
- 1 tablespoon parsley, chopped
- 1 tablespoon feta cheese, crumbled
- Salt and black pepper to the taste

Directions:

1. Heat up your air fryer at 350 degrees F and add oil.
2. Add chorizo and potatoes, stir and brown them for a few seconds.
3. In a bowl, mix eggs with corn, parsley, cheese, salt and pepper and whisk.
4. Pour this over chorizo and potatoes, spread and cook for 5 minutes.
5. Divide omelet on plates and serve for breakfast.

Enjoy!

Nutrition: calories 300, fat 6, fiber 9, carbs 12, protein 6

Egg White Omelet

Preparation time: 10 minutes **Cooking time:** 15 minutes
Servings: 4

Ingredients:

- 1 cup egg whites
- ¼ cup tomato, chopped
- 2 tablespoons skim milk
- ¼ cup mushrooms, chopped
- 2 tablespoons chives, chopped
- Salt and black pepper to the taste

Directions:

1. In a bowl, mix egg whites with tomato, milk, mushrooms, chives, salt and pepper, whisk well and pour into your air fryer's pan.
2. Cook at 320 degrees F for 15 minutes, cool omelet down, slice, divide among plates and serve.

Enjoy!

Nutrition: calories 100, fat 3, fiber 6, carbs 7, carbs 4

Artichoke Frittata

Preparation time: 10 minutes **Cooking time:** 15 minutes
Servings: 6

Ingredients:

- 3 canned artichokes hearts, drained and chopped
- 2 tablespoons olive oil
- ½ teaspoon oregano, dried
- Salt and black pepper to the taste
- 6 eggs, whisked

Directions:

1. In a bowl, mix artichokes with oregano, salt, pepper and eggs and whisk well.
2. Add the oil to your air fryer's pan, add eggs mix and cook at 320 degrees F for 15 minutes.
3. Divide frittata on plates and serve for breakfast.

Enjoy!

Nutrition: calories 136, fat 6, fiber 6, carbs 9, protein 4

Amazing Breakfast Burger

Preparation time: 10 minutes **Cooking time:** 45 minutes
Servings: 4

Ingredients:

- 1 pound beef, ground
- 1 yellow onion, chopped
- 1 teaspoon tomato puree
- 1 teaspoon garlic, minced
- 1 teaspoon mustard
- 1 teaspoon basil, dried
- 1 teaspoon parsley, chopped
- 1 tablespoon cheddar cheese, grated
- Salt and black pepper to the taste
- 4 bread buns, for serving

Directions:

1. In a bowl, mix beef with onion, tomato puree, garlic, mustard, basil, parsley, cheese, salt and pepper, stir well and shape 4 burgers out of this mix.
2. Heat up your air fryer at 400 degrees F, add burgers and cook them for 25 minutes.

3. Reduce temperature to 350 degrees F and bake burgers for 20 minutes more.
4. Arrange them on bread buns and serve for a quick breakfast.

Enjoy!

Nutrition: calories 234, fat 5, fiber 8, carbs 12, protein 4

Onion Frittata

Preparation time: 10 minutes **Cooking time:** 20 minutes
Servings: 6

Ingredients:

- 10 eggs, whisked
- 1 tablespoon olive oil
- 1 pound small potatoes, chopped
- 2 yellow onions, chopped
- Salt and black pepper to the taste
- 1 ounce cheddar cheese, grated
- ½ cup sour cream

Directions:

1. In a large bowl, mix eggs with potatoes, onions, salt, pepper, cheese and sour cream and whisk well.
2. Grease your air fryer's pan with the oil, add eggs mix, place in air fryer and cook for 20 minutes at 320 degrees F.
3. Slice frittata, divide among plates and serve for breakfast.

Enjoy!

Nutrition: calories 231, fat 5, fiber 7, carbs 8, protein 4

Bell Peppers Frittata

Preparation time: 10 minutes **Cooking time:** 20 minutes
Servings: 4

Ingredients:

- 2 tablespoons olive oil
- ½ pounds chicken sausage, casings removed and chopped
- 1 sweet onion, chopped
- 1 red bell pepper, chopped
- 1 orange bell pepper, chopped
- 1 green bell pepper, chopped
- Salt and black pepper to the taste
- 8 eggs, whisked
- ½ cup mozzarella cheese, shredded
- 2 teaspoons oregano, chopped

Directions:

1. Add 1 tablespoon oil to your air fryer, add sausage, heat up at 320 degrees F and brown for 1 minute.
2. Add the rest of the oil, onion, red bell pepper, orange and green one, stir and cook for 2 minutes more.

3. Add oregano, salt, pepper and eggs, stir and cook for 15 minutes.
4. Add mozzarella, leave frittata aside for a few minutes, divide among plates and serve.

Enjoy!

Nutrition: calories 212, fat 4, fiber 6, carbs 8, protein 12

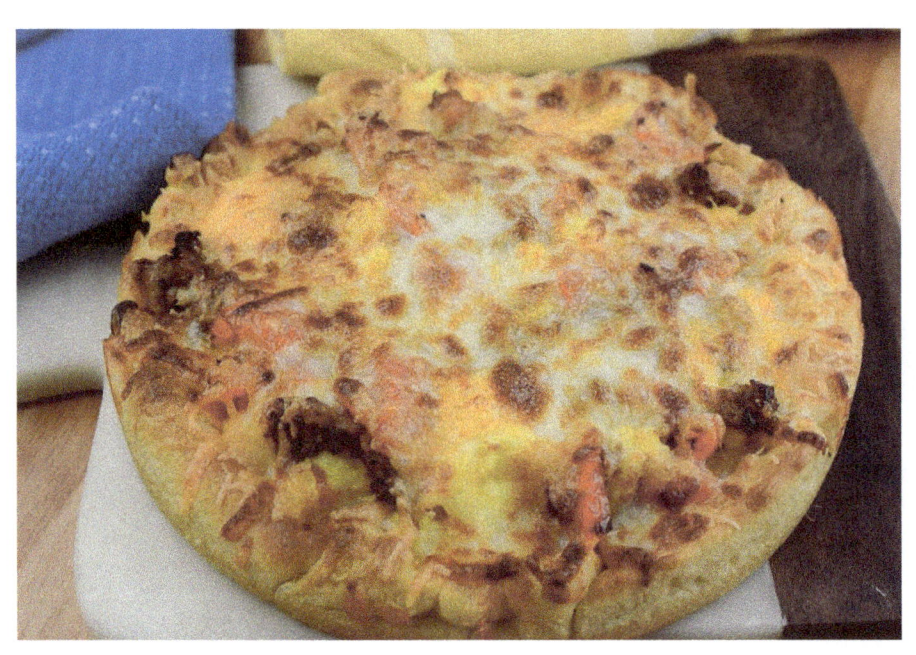

Cheese Sandwich

Preparation time: 10 minutes **Cooking time:** 8 minutes
Servings: 1

Ingredients:

- 2 bread slices
- 2 teaspoons butter
- 2 cheddar cheese slices
- A pinch of sweet paprika

Directions:

1. Spread butter on bread slices, add cheddar cheese on one, sprinkle paprika, top with the other bread slices, cut into 2 halves, arrange them in your air fryer and cook at 370 degrees F for 8 minutes, flipping them once, arrange on a plate and serve.

Enjoy!

Nutrition: calories 130, fat 3, fiber 5, carbs 9, protein 3

Long Beans Omelet

Preparation time: 10 minutes **Cooking time:** 10 minutes
Servings: 3

Ingredients:

- ½ teaspoon soy sauce
- 1 tablespoon olive oil
- 3 eggs, whisked
- A pinch of salt and black pepper
- 4 garlic cloves, minced
- 4 long beans, trimmed and sliced

Directions:

1. In a bowl, mix eggs with a pinch of salt, black pepper and soy sauce and whisk well.
2. Heat up your air fryer at 320 degrees F, add oil and garlic, stir and brown for 1 minute.
3. Add long beans and eggs mix, spread and cook for 10 minutes.
4. Divide omelet on plates and serve for breakfast.

Enjoy!

Nutrition: calories 200, fat 3, fiber 7, carbs 9, protein 3

French Beans and Egg Breakfast Mix

Preparation time: 10 minutes **Cooking time:** 10 minutes
Servings: 3

Ingredients:

- 2 eggs, whisked
- ½ teaspoon soy sauce
- 1 tablespoon olive oil
- 4 garlic cloves, minced
- 3 ounces French beans, trimmed and sliced diagonally
- Salt and white pepper to the taste

Directions:

1. In a bowl, mix eggs with soy sauce, salt and pepper and whisk well.
2. Heat up your air fryer at 320 degrees F, add oil and heat it up as well.
3. Add garlic and brown for 1 minute.
4. Add French beans and egg mix, toss and cook for 10 minutes.
5. Divide among plates and serve for breakfast.

Enjoy!

Nutrition: calories 182, fat 3, fiber 6, carbs 8, protein 3

Breakfast Doughnuts

Preparation time: 10 minutes **Cooking time:** 18 minutes
Servings: 6

Ingredients:

- 4 tablespoons butter, soft
- 1 and ½ teaspoon baking powder
- 2 an ¼ cups white flour
- ½ cup sugar
- 1/3 cup caster sugar
- 1 teaspoon cinnamon powder
- 2 egg yolks
- ½ cup sour cream

Directions:

1. In a bowl, mix 2 tablespoons butter with simple sugar and egg yolks and whisk well.
2. Add half of the sour cream and stir.
3. In another bowls, mix flour with baking powder, stir and also add to eggs mix.
4. Stir well until you obtain a dough, transfer it to a floured working surface, roll it out and cut big circles with smaller ones in the middle.

97

5. Brush doughnuts with the rest of the butter, heat up your air fryer at 360 degrees F, place doughnuts inside and cook them for 8 minutes.
6. In a bowl, mix cinnamon with caster sugar and stir.
7. Arrange doughnuts on plates and dip them in cinnamon and sugar before serving.

Enjoy!

Nutrition: calories 182, fat 3, fiber 7, carbs 8, protein 3

Creamy Breakfast Tofu

Preparation time: 15 minutes **Cooking time:** 20 minutes
Servings: 4

Ingredients:

- 1 block firm tofu, pressed and cubed
- 1 teaspoon rice vinegar
- 2 tablespoons soy sauce
- 2 teaspoons sesame oil
- 1 tablespoon potato starch
- 1 cup Greek yogurt

Directions:

1. In a bowl, mix tofu cubes with vinegar, soy sauce and oil, toss, and leave aside for 15 minutes.
2. Dip tofu cubes in potato starch, toss, transfer to your air fryer, heat up at 370 degrees F and cook for 20 minutes shaking halfway.
3. Divide into bowls and serve for breakfast with some Greek yogurt on the side.

Enjoy!

Nutrition: calories 110, fat 4, fiber 5, carbs 8, protein 4

Veggie Burritos

Preparation time: 10 minutes **Cooking time:** 10 minutes
Servings: 4

Ingredients:

- 2 tablespoons cashew butter
- 2 tablespoons tamari
- 2 tablespoons water
- 2 tablespoons liquid smoke
- 4 rice papers
- ½ cup sweet potatoes, steamed and cubed
- ½ small broccoli head, florets separated and steamed
- 7 asparagus stalks
- 8 roasted red peppers, chopped
- A handful kale, chopped

Directions:

1. In a bowl, mix cashew butter with water, tamari and liquid smoke and whisk well.
2. Wet rice papers and arrange them on a working surface.

3. Divide sweet potatoes, broccoli, asparagus, red peppers and kale, wrap burritos and dip each in cashew mix.

4. Arrange burritos in your air fryer and cook them at 350 degrees F for 10 minutes.

5. Divide veggie burritos on plates d serve.

Enjoy !

Nutrition: calories 172, fat 4, fiber 7, carbs 8, protein 3

Breakfast Fish Tacos

Preparation time: 10 minutes **Cooking time:** 13 minutes
Servings: 4

Ingredients:
- 4 big tortillas
- 1 red bell pepper, chopped
- 1 yellow onion, chopped
- 1 cup corn
- 4 white fish fillets, skinless and boneless
- ½ cup salsa
- A handful mixed romaine lettuce, spinach and radicchio
- 4 tablespoon parmesan, grated

Directions:
1. Put fish fillets in your air fryer and cook at 350 degrees F for 6 minutes.
2. Meanwhile, heat up a pan over medium high heat, add bell pepper, onion and corn, stir and cook for 1-2 minutes.
3. Arrange tortillas on a working surface, divide fish fillets, spread salsa over them, divide mixed veggies

and mixed greens and spread parmesan on each at the end.

4. Roll your tacos, place them in preheated air fryer and cook at 350 degrees F for 6 minutes more.

5. Divide fish tacos on plates and serve for breakfast.

Enjoy!

Nutrition: calories 200, fat 3, fiber 7, carbs 9, protein 5

Garlic Potatoes with Bacon

Preparation time: 10 minutes **Cooking time:** 20 minutes
Servings: 4

Ingredients:

- 4 potatoes, peeled and cut into medium cubes
- 6 garlic cloves, minced
- 4 bacon slices, chopped
- 2 rosemary springs, chopped
- 1 tablespoon olive oil
- Salt and black pepper to the taste
- 2 eggs, whisked

Directions:

1. In your air fryer's pan, mix oil with potatoes, garlic, bacon, rosemary, salt, pepper and eggs and whisk.
2. Cook potatoes at 400 degrees F for 20 minutes, divide everything on plates and serve for breakfast.

Enjoy!

Nutrition: calories 211, fat 3, fiber 5, carbs 8, protein 5

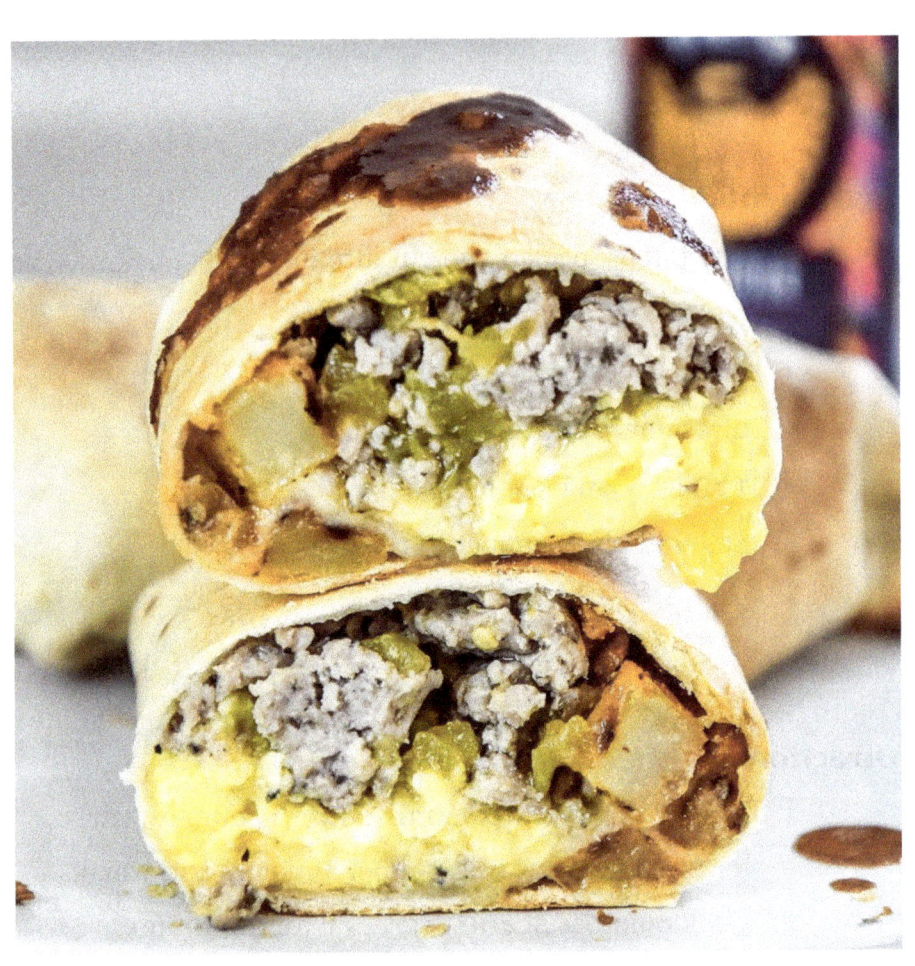

Spinach Breakfast Parcels

Preparation time: 10 minutes **Cooking time:** 4 minutes

Servings: 2

Ingredients:

- 4 sheets filo pastry
- 1 pound baby spinach leaves, roughly chopped
- ½ pound ricotta cheese
- 2 tablespoons pine nuts
- 1 eggs, whisked
- Zest from 1 lemon, grated
- Greek yogurt for serving
- Salt and black pepper to the taste

Directions:

1. In a bowl, mix spinach with cheese, egg, lemon zest, salt, pepper and pine nuts and stir.
2. Arrange filo sheets on a working surface, divide spinach mix, fold diagonally to shape your parcels and place them in your preheated air fryer at 400 degrees F.
3. Bake parcels for 4 minutes, divide them on plates and serve them with Greek yogurt on the side.

Enjoy!

Nutrition: calories 182, fat 4, fiber 8, carbs 9, protein 5

Conclusion

Air frying is one of the most popular cooking methods these days and air fryers have become one of the most amazing tools in the kitchen.
Air fryers help you cook healthy and delicious meals in no time!
You don't need to be an expert in the kitchen in order to cook special dishes for you and your loved ones!
You just have to own an air fryer and this great air fryer cookbook!

You will soon make the best dishes ever and you will impress everyone around you with your home cooked meals!
Just trust us! Get your hands on an air fryer and on this useful air fryer recipes collection and start your new cooking experience! Have fun!

CPSIA information can be obtained
at www.ICGtesting.com
Printed in the USA
BVHW092149220221
600778BV00008B/908